THE VIBRANT BODY

The Simple And Sustainable Way To Feel
Vital And Energised For Life

A.C MILLER

Also by A.C Miller:

The Heartbreak Cure
Reboot

Disclaimer

This book is intended for reference purposes only. The author bears no responsibility for any consequences resulting from the use of information provided in this book. Please use all information at your own risk. Although every effort has been made to ensure factual accuracy, the author is not responsible for any outcome. This book is not a replacement for professional therapy or medical advice. Please seek both of these if you are in need. And please do not stop taking any medication, unless directed by your doctor. If you continue to struggle with your weight or health, or if you feel unwell, please seek professional help as soon as possible.

CONTENTS

INTRODUCTION

This book is going to be short and sweet. The main reason for this is that, over the years, I've read so many books on health, fitness and wellness that seem to confuse rather than enlighten, to complicate rather than simplify. This is why I believe many people are unsuccessful with their goals. Deep down, we know it's a simple formula – more exercise, less unhealthy food. It's not rocket science. Yet there is so much B.S out there, people don't know which way is up.

It's the application of this principle that is hard, not the logic behind it. You KNOW what you need to do, it's just not that easy to make it happen. I know.

I used to eat unhealthily a lot, and ended up putting on quite a bit of weight when I was a student at university. I look back and can see it was mainly a product of drinking beer and eating meat that did it for me. One summer holiday, I made it my mission to lose weight, and ended up on one of those milkshake diets. I hated it. I thought it would be a quick-fix formula and it wasn't. So I lived off Shredded Wheat for a while, and that was also awful. However, I built up some momentum that way, and also started cycling again.

Everything was going well until I moved to Paris.

If you've worked in France before, you'll know that the French get lunch as part of their job perks. Some get a canteen three-course lunch with wine, others (like me) get a lunch voucher. This entitles you to a filled baguette from any local boulangerie, plus a fizzy drink. Oh, and a pastry. Always a pastry. So that was problem number one. Add to that, I developed a strange habit of drinking mojitos after work then eating about five bowls of breakfast cereal when I got home (perhaps a hangover from my Shredded Wheat days). I lived in a tiny shoebox apartment where I'd turn my sofa into a bed each night, but at least meant I could make a cup of tea (or bowl of cereal) without so much as getting up.

I don't know how French women stay so slim because Paris was a disaster for me.

It wasn't until I graduated and went to work on a local radio station that I had a mini epiphany. The week I was there happened to coincide with 'Vegetarian Week' – a week when the Vegetarian Society travel around the UK on a double-decker bus, together with Herb the Dragon, to spread the word about meat-free eating. The timing of this was a huge life blessing for me. I went to interview the Vegetarian Society, armed with a list of questions I'd cobbled together on the train, mostly out of my own prejudices and misinformed ideas, and came away educated and enlightened. Looking back, I was embarrassingly naive, yet these are almost all the same questions I get asked from people today when I talk about food – "Where do you get your protein?", "Humans are supposed to eat meat", "The best way to lose weight is to cut out carbs and live off lean meat". So in a way it was good training.

Needless to say, that week was a seminal moment for me. For the rest of my time at the radio station I compiled my programme on vegetarianism, doing as much research as I could so I could report on the topic with authority. Like most things in life, once you know something, it's very hard to then *unknow* it, and I believe that eating meat was one of those areas where I was loathe to educate myself because then it would mean I'd be obliged to act on that knowledge.

I went veggie for the week of the radio programme to see how it felt and so I could present my findings honestly. And, well, long story short, I never went back. I was genuinely surprised by how different I felt after a week on the veg! The biggest benefit, however, was that I lost weight. This was never the goal, but it was a great byproduct. I always said that if I felt terrible, or if I craved a bacon sandwich (as most people told me I would), I would begin eating meat again. But that never happened. And that was 17 years ago.

Since then, I've continued to ply my trade as a freelance journalist, and over those years I've been lucky enough to work with many top chefs and some of the biggest names in health, fitness and nutrition. I've written a health and food blog, and taken countless courses and retreats around the world in both ancient and cutting-edge medicine and lifestyle choices.

I'm not a qualified nutritionist by any means, but that's not what this book is about. It's a culmination of all the knowledge I've acquired along the way from top sources – knowledge acquired through my own learning, on my own personal journey. And I'm sharing it here because I believe that knowledge may be of value to you, too.

Obesity is one of the biggest killers in the Western world, and the amount of clinically obese people in the UK and US has risen year on year. Doctors consider a person to be obese if they weigh 30% more than the ideal weight for their age, gender and height. Even being overweight by 10-20% can have dire consequences for your health and wellbeing. Yet this is completely avoidable and reversible. So tackling weight head on is THE best thing you can do for yourself, and there's no better time to start than TODAY.

All the things I suggest here have worked for me, and are things I believe will work for you too. Because, ultimately, this book is about being healthy and feeling great, not being skinny or body shaming. If you prefer to lose weight in an extreme, or what I would call 'unsustainable' way, then please go ahead and put this book down now because that's not what this is about. In fact, I'm loathe to even talk about weight loss, since we'll be focusing more on health and wellbeing, and won't be cutting back on food at all – instead switching to different foods altogether – and eating plenty of them, too! This is about taking care of yourself, loving yourself, nurturing yourself, being the best version of yourself, being happy in your own skin.

If you already love the way you look, fantastic. It doesn't matter what size you are, as long as you're happy and healthy. Women especially get bombarded with myriad weight-loss messages, and that in itself is toxic, so that's not what this book is about. What I'm proposing is a way to feel vibrant inside and out. You are what you eat – but you are also the byproduct of the way you think about yourself and treat yourself. Our bodies (and lives) mirror how we think and feel, good and bad. They reflect the words and pictures we play in our heads. Positive body image takes time to cultivate if you've never been used to it, or if you come from parents who also didn't have positive body images. But you don't have to be like your parents – or society, or anyone else, for that matter – and you sure as hell don't have to conform to what the world wants you to look like. You are completely unique and special. This book aims to help you feel much better than you currently do – whatever shape you are.

Some people are afraid to learn about new things because it upsets their version of reality. But that's like staying put and burying your head in the sand. If you want to make any big changes in your life, you've got to be willing to do the work, and, more importantly, put it into practice. Habits are everything. Without educating yourself, you may not reach your destination, and it will take you much longer. So reading and learning about a topic is crucial to making lasting change. Once you educate yourself, it seeps into you on a cellular level. Then it's impossible to turn back.

It's amazing how many people attempt a big lifestyle change without doing any background reading on basic nutrition, cooking or health in general. And that often goes doubly for doctors. I've met many who've given me terrible advice. This is why it's important to take responsibility for your own health and not entrust it into the hands of people who don't know you and your body. You know yourself best. Your health is always YOUR responsibility. Your body is your one and only prize possession. It's the only thing you have for life.

What we know – what has been proven – is that healthy, mindful eating, and regular exercise WORK. It's all about balance, regular routine, and living in harmony with ourselves and with nature. Have too much of anything throws your body out of whack. Do it for too long, and you've upset the delicate balance entirely, often permanently. This is when disease and ill health set in.

This is why most diets don't work – because they're usually extreme. Around 98% of diets fail completely, leading to a loss in motivation and self-esteem. Crash diets can sometimes work for a time, and they can kick-start a healthier eating regime, but they're no good in the long run, and often come with side effects because of their punishing effect on the body and mind. Dieting, by definition, means depriving yourself and pushing your body to extremes. A much better approach is holistic living – mind, body, spirit – and taking it nice and slow. Think about how long it took you to become unhealthy – now think about how long it will take to reverse that damage. So, skip the crash diet altogether and begin here at the beginning – on a more natural road. It will be a longer journey, but a healthier and more mindful one. And your body will thank you for it, I promise.

And remember, there is no rush because you have the rest of your life to do this. But it's important to start today.

Everyone likes to try things once. But standing on the top of a mountain requires you to try again and again, to keep walking and not give up. You've got to get beyond your limited thinking and start making better choices. Choices that will get you to the top of the mountain. As Vince Lombardi said, it's not how many times you fall down, it's how many times you get back up.

I've divided the book into the chapters that I believe make up the most holistic way to lose weight and feel great – food, fitness and feelings, or you could think of it as mind, body and spirit. Food and fitness are all good and well, but without addressing feelings – and getting the way we think about ourselves in check – the whole process is on shaky ground. So the chapter on feelings is a very important one.

We'll look at the emotional and psychological side to eating and being overweight. I will suggest you take up meditation, visualising, goal-setting and journaling. We'll look at tackling root causes to problems, as well as finding joy and meaning in life. Feelings often underpin our life choices in ways we can never truly see until we take the time to examine why we do what we do. The way we feel about ourselves has a drastic impact on how our body looks and feels. By changing those feelings, we can go a long way to becoming truly healthy and getting the body we want and deserve.

The chapter on food will delve into what to eat and what to avoid. I'm going to suggest you stop eating meat and dairy, and, if possible, go completely vegetarian or vegan. But just do as much as you can.

There are myriad reasons for this, which I'll explain later. But essentially I believe this is the healthiest and most sensible way to eat – and one that's best for your body. If it weren't, I wouldn't suggest it. Dining on nothing but steak or protein shakes is what I call a B.S diet. It's B.S for your body, and B.S for the planet. Eating veggie/vegan is the opposite – great for you, great for the planet.

Plus, eating whole foods means you won't need to starve or deprive yourself, so you'll never go hungry. On the contrary, you'll be able to eat much much more, if you want to.

Whenever I hear or read about a new diet, or I talk to someone who's struggling with their weight, I'm always amazed that nobody has suggested to them to just give up meat and dairy. It's so simple to do, makes so much common sense, and is so effective.

Going veggie or vegan is the easiest and most sane way to lose weight, and I'd like you to keep the reasons for it in the forefront of your mind at all times.

In the fitness chapter, I suggest you take up yoga, walking, dancing and cycling. Anything that makes you feel good and doesn't feel like 'exercise'. If you love going to the gym, that's great. You can always add other fitness or sports to the mix – the more the merrier – but yoga, walking (or hiking), dancing and cycling are what have worked well for me – they have low barriers to entry, are simple to start, make you feel on top of the world, and give specific benefits that I'll talk about in this chapter. They're also free.

We'll take a look at the 20% of things that cause us 80% of our problems, and see how we can reduce or eliminate them. Often losing weight can be a good time to shed a few other things, too.

This is a long-term project. I recommend setting aside at least six months of dedicated effort before you expect to see results.

It takes time to break bad habits and build new ones, to make the familiar unfamiliar, and vice versa. Stick with it. A tough patch doesn't last forever, and will be absolutely worth it in the end. Momentum takes a while – and like many things it starts slowly then happens all at once. Think of an aeroplane taking off. Once it's in the air, it can cruise along nicely.

Too many diets focus on the fast-and-furious way to get fit and lose weight. But we all know this isn't ideal, and possibly even dangerous. Rome wasn't built in a day, and all good things come to those who wait. So think long term. And stay positive. The rewards will be yours.

PREPARATION

Preparation is key. It's vital to prepare properly for the coming months to give you the best possible chance of success. If you jump in unprepared, you risk not lasting the distance. You'll need to order the right books and food, research classes, and get organised as you'll be making most of your food from scratch, so you'll need to be ready for this.

Grab a calendar or diary now and do the following:

1. Mark off a date six months in the future as a milestone. This is a realistic goal for looking and feeling very different. Studies now show that it takes 60-100 days to break a habit. Add to that another couple of months to really get going and start to see results. Six months is a good time frame to work towards.

2. Mark off a date three months in the future. This is when you will next weigh yourself. The reason it's so far ahead is that, if you stand on the scales every day (or are in that habit already), it takes your focus off being healthy for the long term. You might gain weight before you lose it, for example, and become disheartened and give up. Or you might gain muscle through your yoga and exercise. By

leaving three months before you weigh yourself again, you shift the focus onto what really matters, and that is your health. You'll know when you've lost weight because of how your body feels, and how your clothes fit, rather than standing on the scales every day.

3. Food shopping. If you can't get to a good supermarket or farm shop regularly, start buying your groceries online. The ideal scenario is to be eating food that is as close to the source as possible – from the ground up. I appreciate this isn't always possible, so the next best thing is to buy organic produce from the supermarket. The next best after that is the fresh produce aisle. Frozen and canned will do, if there's no other choice – but try to mix it with fresh.

   You will also need to bulk-buy items such as brown rice, olive oil, sesame oil, dried fruit, coconut oil, nut butters, nuts, seeds, herbs and spices. I'll talk about this in the food and nutrition chapter, but for now, organise the date when you'll be doing your food shopping so you can stock up on all these items in advance, or know where you can easily source them. Also buy or make sure you have decent food containers as you'll be taking meals with you when you go out to ensure you're eating well even when you're not at home.

4. Research a local yoga class. It's not necessary to attend one because I will show you how you can do a class at home for free, but if you can afford to, it's a good idea to take a class or two at a good yoga centre each week. Not only will this ensure you're doing the postures correctly, but you'll also get to meet new people and have a community who is focused on health.

5. Buy a new bike or get an old one repaired and road-ready.
    There's a lot of scaremongering around cycling, which is a
    great shame because it's a free, easy, healthful way to get
    around. And you get to burn calories and build muscle all
    while getting from A to B and saving money. Research
    cycle paths in your area, and plan routes for where you
    need to go. Riding a bike is strange if you haven't done it
    for years, but as the saying goes, once you're back in the
    saddle, it's like second nature. And I promise that your
    heart, bum and thighs will thank you for it.

6. In your diary or calendar, mark each day that you are
    going to practice yoga and ride your bike. Ideally this will
    be every day, but if you honestly cannot manage that, then
    every other day is fine. But marking it on your calendar
    will ensure it gets done.

7. Buy or take out books on nutrition at your library to
    educate yourself. There is so much misinformation out
    there about basic nutrition, even what we're told by our
    well-meaning parents and teachers can often be wrong.
    Sadly sometimes even by our doctors and healthcare
    professionals. Always do your own research. Buy the
    books I've listed below and read widely around the topics
    covered. Once you start educating yourself on food and
    health, it will be very hard to turn back to the messages we
    blindly inherit from society and other people. Do yourself
    a favour and get the information to educate yourself now.

PART ONE: FOOD

CHAPTER ONE: THE BASICS

———

"Let food be thy medicine." – Hippocrates

Food gets talked about a lot in health and weight loss, but mostly for all the wrong reasons. But food need not be frightening or a source of anxiety. If you eat the right thing! In fact, not all calories are created equal, so I'd like you to forget about them altogether for the time-being. Try also to forget about weighing yourself, and focus instead of the type and quality of food you're putting in your body. Tune into your body and start asking it how it's feeling and what it really wants.

There is one simple way to ensure you're eating the right thing, and that is to eat what your body is asking for then listen to how it responds. How does it feel after eating that food? When you feel great, this is when you know you're eating the right thing for you.

Also, try and eat as close to the source (low on the food chain) as possible. This means:

1. Eating organic whole foods from the land, thus minimising the intake of pesticides and heavy metals, which are more prevalent higher up the food chain.

2. Removing all ready meals, convenience and fast foods, including fizzy drinks, sweets, crisps and so-called 'diet' products.

3. Cutting out – or cutting back on – meat, fish, poultry, eggs and dairy. If you can, go vegetarian or vegan. This will ensure you're eating for optimal nutrition, and takes away much of the stress about what you can and cannot eat. If you've bought a good vegetarian or vegan cookbook, simply work your way through it, enjoying all the new flavours and recipes, safe in the knowledge that you're eating a diet that will not only help you lose weight, but help you live longer and become healthier in general.

4. Eating as much whole, fresh plant-based produce as you can – fruits, vegetables, nuts and seeds. You'll never go hungry because you will have so much wonderful food to eat!

5. Reducing sugar, salt and fat intake – olive oil, sesame oil, coconut, walnut and flax oils are fine. Make sure they are organic and cold-pressed, and that you store them in your fridge.

6. Reducing alcohol intake – or taking a break from it altogether and switching to green tea or herbal teas.

7. Eating regular small meals – five smaller meals instead of three large ones, for example. This stops you feeling neither hungry nor bloated, maintains your blood sugar

levels, and means you get a steady stream of nutrients and energy throughout the day.

8. Eating until you're 80% full – ie, stopping before you 'feel full'. Let the food go down and see how you feel then. Let your stomach empty before you fill it again. If you eat a nutrient-rich, whole-foods diet, you can do very well on 1,500 calories a day.

9. If you really need to snack, make sure you have plenty of fresh fruit, nuts and vegetables to hand (carrying them with you, if necessary), though try to get used to not eating between meals.

10. Drink plenty of water – aim for at least two litres a day, and stop drinking after dinner to give yourself enough time to eliminate liquid before going to sleep. The other drink I recommend is green tea. This can be matcha (powdered green tea), jasmine or white tea, and can be taken hot or cold. In fact, it's good to have a jug of cold green tea in the fridge to sip on throughout the day, as well as drinking it hot in a mug. Green tea is full of antioxidants and is extremely good for you[1]. So ditch all fizzy drinks entirely, and substitute them with green tea and water instead.

If you really can't or don't want to cut out meat and dairy, reduce your consumption to the absolute minimal amounts, and ensure these come from responsible sources. But try and eat as much fruit, vegetables, nuts and seeds as possible so that these make up the bulk of your diet, then have the odd bit of animal produce if

---

[1] https://nutritionfacts.org/video/can-green-tea-help-prevent-cancer/

you really need to. If you eat all of the foods I suggest in this chapter, it will be hard to find room for meat products anyway, unless you have a colossal appetite, and remember, we're only eating until we're 80% full, so stuffing in that grilled chicken breast will be up to your better judgement.

If you really, really cannot give up meat, you could always eat vegetarian or vegan during the week, and eat meat at the weekend and see how both make you feel, then decide from there what's best for you. The important thing is to tune into your body and work out the foods that serve it best and allow it to be fully healthy and able to heal itself.

Why do I suggest you go vegetarian or vegan to lose weight and be healthy?

1. Studies that compare the diets of meat-eaters with flexitarians, pescetarians, vegetarians and vegans show that it's the latter group who are the slimmest, with an average BMI of 23.6. Meat-eaters have an average BMI of 28.8[2].

2. A whole-food, plant-based diet has been proven in scientific studies to prevent, and often reverse some of the world's biggest killers – heart disease, high cholesterol, type-2 diabetes and high blood pressure. Plant-based diets are naturally cholesterol free, high in fibre, and have also been shown to control weight and blood sugar levels[3], give you cleaner arteries, improve sleep quality, mental health[4] and emotional states, and ease depression, anxiety

---

[2] https://nutritionfacts.org/topics/weight-loss

[3] https://nutritionfacts.org/topics/plant-based-diets/

[4] https://nutritionfacts.org/video/plant-based-diets-for-improved-mood-and-

and fatigue. An all-round win-win.

3. On the flip side, meat and dairy can cause inflammation, high cholesterol, high blood pressure, diabetes, clogged arteries and heart disease. The nitrates in bacon have been linked to cancer[5]. Fried meat can cause rancidity, which can also lead to cancer. Hormones, pesticides, antibiotics and other toxins pass from meat and dairy into our bodies and cause us untold harm, so cutting them out of your diet eliminates the risk of this unnecessary toxic load.

    A lot of conventionally produced meat and dairy comes from animals reared in stressful conditions, and often these animals are fed growth-stimulating hormones or *other animals* that weren't fit for human consumption, yet still end up in the food chain as animal feed.

    I'm not sure why anyone would want to do this to their own body when there is so much other good food to eat, with minimal risk of disease and harm for us or the environment, but if you still wish to eat meat and dairy, try and buy organic and free-range products from local farmers or a reputable supermarket or butcher. Personally I don't think the risk is worth it, but this is your own choice.

4. Whole, plant-based diets lead to better digestion and an increase in productivity, vitality and energy (exactly what we need when we're trying to lose weight)[6]. The myth that

---

productivity/
[5]https://www.theguardian.com/news/2018/mar/01/bacon-cancer-processed-meats-nitrates-nitrites-sausages
[6] https://nutritionfacts.org/topics/plant-based-diets/

vegetarians and vegans lack energy doesn't hold water when you learn how to eat properly and feed your body nutrient-dense foods. The word 'vegetarian' comes from the Latin 'vegetabilis', which means lively or animated, which is how a vegetarian diet makes you feel. If you're feeling lethargic and depleted, you're not eating right. This is why it's important to educate yourself on basic nutrition.

5. By minimising or eliminating meat, you have more room for fruits and vegetables, never feel hungry and STILL lose weight! Even if you did nothing else after reading this book except add more fruit and vegetables to your diet (while still eating exactly the same as before), you would lose weight and feel better. But why not just switch to different foods completely and enjoy the full benefits of a plant-based diet?[7] If you go completely vegan for three weeks, you can decide for yourself whether it's worth continuing or not. Three weeks out of your life isn't much.

6. A low-fat, high-fibre, plant-based diet can save you money, if you know how to shop wisely[8]. If you bulk buy your store cupboard items such as brown and basmati rice, beans, lentils, nuts, seeds, oils, herbs and spices, and you buy your fruits and vegetables organic and fresh, and you remove meat, dairy and fish from your list, your grocery costs should be greatly reduced. It's a myth that eating healthily costs money. Nearly all of the lower-income and developing countries I've visited, where a large portion of the population earn less than a dollar a day, live off whole

---

[7] Eat More to Weigh Less, https://nutritionfacts.org/video/eating-more-to-weigh-less/

[8] https://nutritionfacts.org/video/superfood-bargains-2/

foods and fresh vegetables – mostly homegrown. Meat is
a luxury they often cannot afford.

Think of all the wonderful meat-free dishes found in India,
Thailand, Mexico, Morocco, Turkey, Greece, China and
Japan? It's really a case of educating yourself on what to
buy and how to cook it. An education that will pay
dividends for your health and bank balance in the long run[9].
 Check out the Vegan Society's blog for more inspiration
on budget recipes from around the world[10].

---

[9] The Cost of a Vegan Diet: https://www.vegansociety.com/whats-
new/blog/cost-vegan-diet-international-perspective
[10] https://www.vegansociety.com/resources/recipes/budget

CHAPTER TWO: SO WHAT *CAN* I EAT?

Pretty much most fresh, natural produce. Beans, legumes, fruits, vegetables, seeds and other plants – making sure they're organic to minimise pesticide and toxic load. You want to eat things that are alive and bursting with vitality because that's the effect they will have on you! Dead foods – food that has been sitting around for days on a shelf, or which has travelled far or been sprayed with all manner of preservatives – will make us feel dead, too. Even if you don't "like" fruit and veg, treat it as medicine – you don't have to enjoy it for it to be doing you the power of good. That said, not all plants are created equal.

Here I've outlined some of the most nutritionally dense plant foods, so if all you do is eat from this list, you'll be healthier and lighter in no time. Not only will eating these kinds of foods help you lose weight, and therefore live longer, a lot of them have been proven to aid longevity and fight disease in their own right, too. So it's a double whammy.

And as for feeling hungry – quite the opposite! You'll struggle to work your way through all the items on this list each day.

As I mentioned in the chapter on preparation, once you've ordered all your fresh produce and bulk-bought your rice, flour, oils etc, all you need to do is experiment putting it all together. You can make smoothies, juices, salads, soups, stews, curries, breads, dips – the list is endless. I've included a couple of ideas below, but the best thing is to buy a decent recipe book and experiment with whatever you fancy.

Soup

Soup is healthy, nutritious and filling. It's also cheap to make. Make a fresh batch of soup once or twice a week and freeze or refrigerate it so you can enjoy a bowl every day. It's shown in studies that those who eat a bowl of soup a day lose more weight than those who don't, but eat the same number of calories[11] – so get souping! Soup is extremely easy to make – have a look at the Vegan Planet recipe book for some ideas. How about a Thai-style coconut soup? A Cuban black-bean soup? A spicy lentil dahl? The choices are endless.

Juices and salads

Raw food has so many health benefits, as well as making you feel alive and energised. Try and get at least half your fruit and vegetable intake from raw sources. Maybe have a salad each lunchtime, or a salad before each meal to get some raw nutrients into your system. Grab a copy of *Becoming Raw* or *The Raw Foods Bible* and give them a thorough read. You could try having one day a week of eating raw or drinking fruit and vegetable juice to give your digestive system a break. Make sure you drink plenty of water if you do this, and get plenty of rest.

Oil and fats

Flax, extra-virgin olive, walnut, sesame and almond oils all contain Omega-3 essential fatty acids and GLA (gamma linolenic acid), which is crucial for brain and heart health, good skin, and a functioning immune system. These are what you'll be cooking and dressing your salads with. Try and buy organic, cold-pressed

---

[11] Secrets of Longevity by Dr Maoshing Ni

oils, and as best you can, stay away from margarine, sunflower oil and butter. And definitely no deep-fat-frying!

Herbs and spices

One of the biggest complaints I hear levelled against a non-meat 'diet' is that it's boring or tasteless. Nothing could be further from the truth, and I'm sorry that has been your experience so far. Vegan food has to be some of the tastiest food on the planet, making the most of the wonderful fresh produce we have access to, as well as spicing it up for extra flavour and health benefits.

Herbs and spices are very good for you, so go ahead and make that curry/stir-fry/soup/casserole! Turmeric has been used as an anticoagulant in Asia for centuries – it also reduces inflammation and can help ward off certain cancers. Aim for half a teaspoon of ordinary powdered turmeric a day, which can be added to soups and curries – or smoothies (you don't taste it!).

Broccoli

Broccoli is the wonder veg. It has so much nutritional value, it's hard to beat. Also, per calorie, it has more protein than beef, and contains cancer-fighting properties, amino acids, fibre and vitamin B6. Out of all the cruciferous vegetables, broccoli produces the highest amount of antioxidant and anti-carcinogen **sulforaphane**. Sulforaphane helps our liver detoxify pollution, and studies have shown it also helps reduce the risk of lung cancer – and even inhibit its progress[12].

Try to eat it fresh (not frozen) every day. You can eat it raw, but if you prefer to cook it, chop it up and leave it for 45 minutes first. Or add half a teaspoon of mustard powder or mustard seeds,

---

[12] Lung Cancer Metastases and Lung Cancer:
https://nutritionfacts.org/video/lung-cancer-metastases-and-broccoli/

which keeps all the benefits of raw broccoli even when it's cooked or frozen[13]. Then you can steam it or roast it and drizzle with olive oil and a few sea-salt flakes or Tahini dressing, or enjoy it *au naturale*.

Other green leafy cruciferous vegetables to eat plenty of include cauliflower, cabbage, bok choy, brussels sprouts, kale, collard greens, watercress, rutabaga, wasabi, arugula and radish – all these have potential anti-cancer effects[14], as well as sulforaphane for detoxification[15].

Vegetables

Fruit and vegetables are the most nutritionally dense foods available – particularly green leafy veg, which top the charts of nutrients. So the world is your lobster (or veg patch) here. You can eat as many fresh vegetables as you like, and experiment with how to cook them.

My personal preference is to roast peppers, aubergine, beetroot and garlic and add some braised mushrooms to the mix. These can be eaten with jacket potatoes, roasted sweet potatoes, made into curries or stews, or added to sandwiches. As long as you always have plenty of this mix in the fridge, you'll never reach for an unhealthy alternative.

Always make sure you have a stockpile of broccoli, sweet potatoes, baking potatoes, butternut squash, onions, garlic, peppers, carrots, courgettes, aubergine, tomatoes, bok choy, spinach, sweetcorn, artichoke, cauliflower, asparagus, pumpkin,

---

[13] https://nutritionfacts.org/video/second-strategy-to-cooking-broccoli/

[14] Breast cancer survival vegetable: https://nutritionfacts.org/video/breast-cancer-survival-vegetable/

[15] https://www.livestrong.com/article/307835-foods-that-are-high-in-sulforaphane/

beetroot. Spinach is 50% protein and full of iron and vitamin C[16] so add it to your salads and green smoothies.

Preparation is key here – do all your chopping and cooking in one fell swoop to save time. Then you can cook as you go. Or roast a big batch, then dip into it throughout the coming days. You can also enjoy many of these raw – as crudites dipped in hummus, as raw vegetable juice, soup or coleslaw.

Mushrooms

Technically a fungus not a plant, mushrooms' nutritional and healing properties are quite extraordinary, and we're still learning about their far-reaching applications even now. Suffice it to say that this food group should be high on your list of what to eat. Mushrooms contain a substance called **ergothioneine**, which is a natural amino acid (a building block for protein) and which has antioxidant, anti-ageing, anti-cancer and anti-UV qualities, among others. It doesn't matter too much which mushrooms you buy, though organic is always preferable. I'd be cautious about picking your own unless you are 110% certain you know what you're doing. Mushrooms can be deadly in only small amounts.

Beans, lentils, garden peas, chickpeas and tempeh

Try and include these in as many meals as you can. You can add them to soups and stews and salads, or blend them into pates or hummus (try the recipes below), and use raw carrots and peppers to dip into it. Beans include pinto, butter beans, kidney beans, edamame and cannellini and black beans. Soybeans are a complete protein, meaning that they contain all nine essential amino acids. This makes them a great alternative to meat.

---

[16]http://www.onegreenplanet.org/natural-health/soy-free-vegan-foods-that-have-more-protein-than-beef/

Berries

Red, purple and blue berries contain anthocyanin flavonoids, which are anti-inflammatory and antioxidant. Blueberries, in particular, have the highest levels of these flavonoids and have been shown to slow down the signs of ageing and protect the brain from age-related memory loss and plaque. But you can add these to any other combination of berries to make a rich smoothie – try acai, goji, blackberries (pick them when in season and freeze for later use), strawberries, raspberries and cranberries. Blend with apple juice, cold green tea, ground flax seeds and a pinch of turmeric for an anti-ageing, anti-inflammatory, kick-ass smoothie.

Apples

An apple a day really does keep the doctor away. Not only has apple peel been linked to reducing certain types of cancers, but eating an apple before your meal will make you feel less hungry, and their fibre will bind with the fat molecules to reduce fat absorption. So eat at least an apple a day – preferably three!

Beetroot

Fresh, raw beetroot is good for juicing and grating over salads. You can also chop it and boil it or roast it and add it to your roasted veg mix. Containing folate, which is necessary for healthy cells, and full of vitamins, minerals and anti-carcinogens, it's almost unrivalled in terms of its nutritional value – you can also use its tops in salads and soups, just like spinach. A beetroot, carrot and fresh apple juice (ABC juice) is an excellent way to consume this root vegetable.

Sea vegetables

Arame, dulse, nori, kombu, kelp and Irish moss contain more micronutrients than land vegetables and are believed to have life-extending and life-enhancing properties. Seaweed, for example, contains more calcium, iron and protein than meat or dairy.

Whales only eat single-cell organisms called plankton, yet are the biggest mammals on the planet.

Freshwater single-cell algae such as **chlorella,** and cyanobacteria such as **spirulina,** contain the highest source of protein of any foodstuff – 58.4% compared with beef's 52% – as well as being an excellent vegan source of iron[17]. Chlorella contains the highest source of chlorophyll of any plant. Wheatgrass juice is a good source of chlorophyll, or you can take chlorella and spirulina tablets or powder as a supplement.

Nuts and seeds

Nuts and seeds should make up a considerable portion of your daily food. Containing protein, potassium, phosphorus, calcium, iron, copper, and most of the B vitamins, they're an excellent substitute for meat. Nuts contain **good fats**, and are also one of the best plant-based sources of vitamin E.

Arginine – a non-essential amino acid found in nuts and seeds – helps fight disease and stimulate the pituitary gland, which releases all-important growth hormones needed for healing.

Flaxseeds contain Omega-3 and 6 essential fatty acids, and perform remarkably well in studies to reduce blood pressure.

But perhaps their crowning glory is that they contain more than 100 times more anti-cancerous **lignans** than *any other foods*, making them the richest known source of this potent anti-carcinogen. They're particularly helpful in fighting breast and prostate cancers[18].

---

[17] https://www.bbcgoodfood.com/howto/guide/health-benefits-spirulina
[18] https://nutritionfacts.org/topics/flax-seeds

Hemp seeds are also fantastic – full of protein, magnesium and omega 3 and 6 fatty acids. They can also help boost your metabolism, so are great when losing weight[19]. Stir into your morning oatmeal, or add to your smoothies.

Nuts are an amazing source of protein. In fact, one pound of walnuts has the equivalent food value of four pounds of red meat and 10 pounds of chicken. An acre of walnuts will supply more than 1,000 pounds of 'shelled meats', with a food value of 3,000,000 calories – 20 times the amount the same acre would yield in beef.[20]

Because they're so nutrient-dense, you only need 7-9 walnuts a day. Keep a bag of your own mixed nut and seed blend in your bag to munch on throughout the day. Try cashews, almonds (see below), flax, pumpkin seeds, pine kernels, chia seeds, brazil nuts and hemp seeds. Also stock up on (or make your own) nut butters – peanut, cashew, almond, hazelnut and tahini can all be spread on oat cakes or toast for a tasty high-protein snack.
Almonds are particularly good to eat when you're trying to lose weight because they contain high levels of unsaturated fats that can lower cholesterol and even reduce the risk of heart disease. Although almonds aren't low in calories or fat, calories and fats are not created equal, and can be good or bad. In almonds it's all good. So snack away! Particularly at night, as almonds contain magnesium, which relaxes your muscles and helps you sleep, and tryptophan, which helps your body produce sleep hormone melatonin. You can also make your own almond milk, almond hummus (see below) and almond butter, and enjoy these spread on bagels, oat cakes or rye bread for a protein-rich snack[21]. If you

---

[19]http://www.onegreenplanet.org/natural-health/soy-free-vegan-foods-that-have-more-protein-than-beef/
[20] Vegetarianism: Green Grow the Dishes by HTV

carry around a bag of almonds you'll never go hungry because you can always dip into them as necessary.

WARNING:
Beware of eating immature almonds, which have softer, greener shells. These can contain a compound that produces hydrogen cyanide. Children under four, and pregnant or breastfeeding mothers, should avoid peanuts. And store all nuts in cool, dry place to avoid mould.

Whole grains
Brown and basmati rice, brown bread, oats, barley, quinoa – eating whole grains ensures a good intake of fibre and protein, and a steady source of energy. This makes it good for weight loss as you feel fuller for longer as your blood sugar is kept more constant.

In one randomised control trial, consuming just three portions of whole grains a day was found to "significantly reduce" the risk of heart disease in middle-aged people, and believed to be as powerful as high-blood-pressure medication in reducing hypertension[22]. Oats and barley are even more powerful, and lower your cholesterol too!

Rice constitutes half of the world's staple diet. Much of its nutritional value is stored in the germ and bran, so brown rice is better for you than white, which has actually been linked to type-2 diabetes[23]. So stick to brown, if you can. Basmati is also good for losing weight.

---

[21] http://www.onegreenplanet.org/natural-health/soy-free-vegan-foods-that-have-more-protein-than-beef/

[22] https://bit.ly/2K3g7bT

[23] https://nutritionfacts.org/video/whole-grains-may-work-as-well-as-drugs/

Make up a big batch of brown rice and quinoa (which is protein dense at 14%), then keep this in the fridge or freezer so you can scoop a portion into a bowl and eat with one of your veggie curries, soups or stews, or your simple roast veg mix.

As bread is one of the most processed products we can buy, it makes sense to make your own so you know what goes in it. It's cheaper too. Don't be put off by the time it takes to make bread as a lot of it consists of leaving the bread alone to 'prove', which can be done overnight. As with everything in this book, it's about planning and setting yourself up for success rather than buckle at the first hurdle or sniff of hard work. Bread takes time. All good things take time. That's just life. Baking homemade bread is one of the greatest, and simplest, pleasures. *Enjoy it.*

Brown bread is so easy to make – you simply mix together 520g of whole wheat flour, a pinch of sea salt and a packet of instant yeast (11g). Then add 480ml warm water into which you've dissolved 2 tsp of agave syrup or raw honey. Once the mixture is combined, tip it into a greased bread tin, cover with a clean tea towel and leave to prove for as long as you like (at least half an hour, though overnight is best). Bake in a 200C oven for 30-40 mins and leave to cool before tipping onto a rack or tin.

You could also try making seed bread, which is a great way of ensuring you get all your daily quota of seeds. Drizzle toasted slices of this amazing creation with olive oil, add mashed avocado or homemade hummus, and life is golden.

Basic hummus recipe

___

1 x 400g can of chickpeas
1 garlic clove, peeled and chopped
1 tbsp Tahini
Juice of 1 lemon
Extra virgin olive oil

Drain the chickpeas and add to a food processor with the garlic, Tahini, lemon juice and 1 tbsp of olive oil. Add a pinch of sea salt and blitz until smooth. Taste to check seasoning and consistency, and add more salt, lemon or water as required. Serve with a drizzle of olive oil.

___

Almond hummus recipe

___

500g blanched or flaked almonds
600g water
Juice of 2 lemons
1 garlic clove, peeled and chopped
50g sherry vinegar
2 tsp ground cumin
1 tsp paprika
½ tsp chilli powder (to taste)
½ tsp cayenne powder
1 tsp nutritional yeast
1 tsp soy sauce
600g extra virgin olive oil

Toast the almonds at 180 C until browned. Once cool, add to the
blender or bullet and blitz with all the other ingredients except the
oil. Drizzle in the oil slowly until the desired consistency is
formed. Taste and season with sea salt and freshly ground black
pepper to taste.

TOP TIP:
Place extra portion-sized quantities of the dried ingredients into
food bags, together with the toasted almonds, so you're ready to
make your next batch at a moment's notice.

CHAPTER THREE: PROTEIN

I'm including a chapter on protein because it's a word I hear bandied around a lot, with little understanding of what it actually means.

Protein gets so much air time in the West, and we're conditioned to believe that we're somehow lacking and we need to consume vast quantities of it. We're also conditioned to believe that the best way to do this is to eat lots of meat. Both these beliefs are simply not true. If you think about it, elephants, whales, rhino, giraffe, horses, cattle, hippo and gazelles get all the protein they need from a plant-based diet – mostly by eating grass or hay – and they're not exactly weak and feeble creatures. Nor are they overweight, for that matter.

The average adult needs around 0.8 grams of protein per kilogram of body weight. To find out how much protein you need, multiply your average weight in pounds by 0.36, then double the answer. It's widely accepted that the average male needs around 56 grams, and the average female 46 grams of protein a day. Add a bit more if you're pregnant, breast-feeding, elderly or very active.

So why are humans so obsessed with protein, and with getting it from meat?

Mostly this comes down to social conditioning, and the concept of meat and blood symbolising strength and power. Masai warriors used to drink the blood of a lion to give them courage.

Protein and meat are linked in most people's minds – protein, meat, strength and muscle.

But let's unpick this a second.

Proteins are needed in the body to build muscle and tissue – yes. And meat is a 'complete protein' – correct. However, a complete protein can also be found in quinoa, spirulina, soybeans and buckwheat (just as an example).

So what exactly are proteins? Proteins are like strings of beads made up of amino acids. Most of these amino acids can be made by the body. Only nine cannot, and these are called **essential amino acids** and need to be obtained from food. Foods known as 'complete proteins' contain all nine of these essential amino acids. Complete proteins include meat, dairy and eggs, quinoa, chlorella, spirulina and soybeans.

However – and this is really important to understand – even so-called 'incomplete proteins' can, at the end of the day, be combined by your body to give you all the amino acids and protein you need.

So there really is no need to worry about consuming 'complete' proteins at all!

If you eat a varied diet of plant produce, over the course of the day your body tallies it all up and makes the full amount of amino acids (thus protein) it needs. There. Easy.

What are some good plant sources of protein? Chlorella and spirulina (around 58% – which is far more than meat), spinach (51%), peanuts (26%), almonds (21%), kidney beans (24%), pinto beans (21%), pumpkin seeds (19%), flaxseeds (18%), oats (17%), wheat (12.6%), chickpeas (9%), lentils (9%), quinoa (14%), chia (16.5%), sorghum (10.6%), and barley (12%)[24]. In many developing countries these food groups are combined to great effect.

If you think about it, when we were hunter gatherers, we often went long periods without meat. Even lions and tigers aren't always successful on a hunt. We're lucky in that we can survive just as well with or without meat. And in the 21st-century Western world, we're hardly lacking in options. It really is about choice – and education.

At the moment, there is no known protein deficiency in Western cultures. Moreover – and this is a vital point to make – many people in Western societies actually consume ***too much* protein**[25]. Eating too much protein can damage your heart, kidneys and bones, and lead to osteoporosis. In fact, osteoporosis is caused more by protein excess than calcium deficiency. The rate of osteoporosis in America is higher than that of China, where most people eat a low-protein vegetarian diet.[26] Consuming too much protein means you have to get rid of excess nitrogen from your blood, which stresses out your kidneys, and dehydrates your body.

So – in short – yes, we need protein, but we don't need to consume so much of it, nor 'complete proteins' at every meal, and definitely not from meat. We can eat 'incomplete proteins' from plenty of other plant sources, and still make up our protein quota

---

[24]http://www.onegreenplanet.org/natural-health/soy-free-vegan-foods-that-have-more-protein-than-beef/

[25] Proteinaholic by Garth Davis MD, http://proteinaholic.com/

[26] Secrets of Longevity by Dr Maoshing Ni

for the day. Just think about racehorses the next time you question where you get your protein from.

CALCIUM

Yet another Western fallacy. We do not need to consume vast quantities of milk or cheese to get calcium and build our bones. We can get ample supplies of calcium from plant sources, and therefore reduce our risk of osteoporosis without consuming too much protein. Tofu and other soy products, green leafy vegetables, nuts and seeds (especially sesame), dried fruits (especially figs), blackstrap molasses, broccoli and sea vegetables are all excellent sources of calcium, all without the risk of nasty diseases or weight gain.

IRON

We need iron to make red blood cells and haemoglobin, which carries oxygen to our tissues. Although vegetable sources of iron – such as green leafy vegetables, lentils, nuts and dried fruits – aren't as easily absorbed as animal sources, combining them with fresh fruit or a glass of orange juice helps the body get all the iron it needs.

VITAMIN B12

When you remove meat and dairy from your diet, it's important to get your vitamin B12 from other sources. Fortified foods, such as breakfast cereal, contain B12, though the best supply if you're trying to lose weight is soy milk and nutritional yeast (brewer's yeast). You can also take a supplement, if you prefer. You only need 2 micrograms of B12 a day, and our bodies can store and recycle it for years, so you really don't need to worry about becoming deficient. I hope that has dispelled some of the myths about basic nutrition.

CHAPTER FOUR: DETOXIFICATION

To keep your body in its healthiest, most vibrant form, try to do a cleanse at least once a year. Spring is a good time to do this. There are various ways to cleanse the body, but my preferred method is a combination of food and herbs. Take a look at *The Cure For All Diseases* by Hulda Regehr Clark for more detailed information.

1. **DIET**: Do as many days as you can. Even two days are better than none. But ideally you want to do two weeks. Try and eat only organic fruits and vegetables – either juiced, raw or cooked.

2. **HERBS:** Take a herbal tincture for a parasite cleanse. Our bodies are always picking up parasites, flukes and worms, and this is the underlying cause of many diseases and illnesses. You can buy a ready-made tincture of three herbs from a company called Nature's Answer (make sure it's the 2,000mg strength), which you take first thing in the morning on an empty stomach, then again after lunch, and once more before bed. Or you can buy each herb separately and mix your own. The herbs are: black walnut hull tincture extra strength (2 tsp dose), wormwood (1-2ml doses) and freshly ground cloves (500mg doses). Also take milk thistle and ornithine each night before bed, and 500mg of L-arginine in the morning after breakfast. Plus 1,000mg of vitamin C. Continue this for 10-14 days then take a break for a week before continuing for another 10-14 days. Then throughout the year, take a maintenance dose once a week.

PART TWO: FITNESS

CHAPTER FOUR: YOGA

If you want to lose weight, you'll need to combine aerobic activity (cardio) with anaerobic activity – things that strengthen and build muscle. Yoga can do both.

The reason I suggest taking up yoga is that it's possibly the best all-round health practice I know of. I'd say my second epiphany, after I gave up meat, was discovering yoga. Amazingly, we were actually taught yoga in primary school, but it wasn't until I was 26 that I started a regular practice. I bought the AM:PM DVD on Amazon and would follow each routine morning and night in my bedroom. It was a game-changer. I couldn't afford to go to a class in London, so this was brilliant for me. My body made a complete and fundamental shift from that point forth. This was years before the dawn of YouTube and all the free and incredible yoga resources you can find online, and definitely pre-Instagram yoga gods and goddesses striking poses on tropical beaches. And thank goodness! The yoga I learned had nothing to do with looking hot in Lycra, and everything to do with personal inner journey.

More than just a series of poses or stretches, yoga is a whole integrated system of psychological, spiritual and physical wellbeing. The more you practice, the more it transforms your body and mind in very subtle but noticeable ways. Yoga eliminates toxins and stimulates healing. It also helps you feel grounded and calm, with a renewed sense of self. To say it's ideal for health is an understatement.

And for every hour of yoga you do, you also get an hour of meditation and relaxation thrown in for good measure!

Regularly practicing yoga tones up the muscles and, as muscle tissue burns more calories than body fat, even when you're resting, it's great for losing weight.

Yoga also helps you tune into your body, and zone out from the stresses of everyday life. When you're on the mat, nothing else seems to matter. It forces you to look inward instead of outside yourself and is very calming and rejuvenating.

Don't worry if you've never done it before, or don't feel 'flexible enough' – everybody has to start somewhere. You get flexible by practicing the yoga, that's the point. Imagine if you had the same attitude towards walking or riding a bike! You'd be a couch potato. And never, ever compare yourself with other people in your class because they all started at the beginning too, and this is your own personal journey, not theirs.

Yoga means 'yoke' or 'union' in Sanskrit, and it seeks to unite the body and mind with the greater consciousness. The postures (or asanas) are just one part of the whole system – just one of the eight 'limbs' of yoga – so don't be put off if you find them difficult to begin with. They're there for a reason, and that is to prepare your mind for meditation, which you hopefully get to enjoy at the end of the session. If you feel impatient, irritated, stressed, tense or inflexible, this is *precisely* why you need to be doing yoga – please remember that!
Take your time to try out different classes and teachers to find one that suits you best. Not all yoga teachers are created equal, so it's important you find the right fit for you. And the bonus is you will meet lots of lovely people, too.

If you can't get to a class, or it's too expensive to take one (and unfortunately they can be), there are lots of free yoga videos on Youtube. My personal favourite is Yoga With Adriene (link in the resources section). You can also still buy the AM:PM DVD with Patricia Walden – it's not free, but once you've bought it, you'll have it for life. It was a great introduction for me, and I'm sure will be for you too. You can always take a class in person once a week, just to make sure you're getting your asanas and alignment right, then do the online classes at home in between – this is what I do and it works very well.

A key part of yoga is BREATHING (or pranayama). This is deceptively simple but hugely effective, if learned properly. Yoga breathing is done through the nose – and I recommend you always breathe through the nose, even when not doing yoga. This provides the body with more oxygen and cleans the air. It also helps shape the face and teeth. Have a look at the Buteyko breathing method: (www.buteykoclinic.com) and Patrick McKeown's work. You can also look at the Wim Hof method of breathing (www.wimhofmethod.com), which is a more intense form of pranayama (yogic breathing). Controlling the breath is one of the fastest and most powerful ways to health and wellbeing.

Namaste!

CHAPTER FIVE: WALKING

———————

"Sitting is the new smoking."

Walking will fall into your 'aerobic/cardio activity' camp because it increases your heart rate and gets the blood pumping. Research also shows that taking a long walk each day reduces stress and boosts mental health, all of which will help you to feel better and sleep better. Amen!

Walking is free and easy and should make up a large portion of your daily exercise. If you don't have the time to take a long walk each day, think about how you can incorporate a walk into your daily commute – possibly by walking to work? Or walking at least one of the journeys. You could also take a walk in your lunch break.

Walking is great for mental health. When we're walking, we have time to think and formulate proper thoughts and ideas. Too much of our modern lives is spent sat in front of a screen of some sort, and this is bad for both our bodies and minds. Getting out in nature and taking a good walk helps sort out your head as well as your heart. Just as I like to think of food as plant medicine, I like to think of walking as movement medicine.

My personal favourite is to take a walk first thing in the morning before I do anything else – definitely before checking emails or social media. I get up, splash my face, take a sip of water, then hit the road. This really helps set me up for the day, gives my lungs a boost of oxygen, my skin a boost of vitamin D, and my mind time to wake up. I still feel my brain is in dream/creative mode, so it's a great time to be thinking about 'bigger picture' stuff. It's also when I get clarity on what I need to be doing that day, and in life in general – sorting out what's important, and what's not. When I'm walking I usually ask myself "What's the most important thing I need to do today?" – then as soon as I get back home, I get on it.

There are plenty of apps out there to help you measure how far you've walked each day, and how many calories you've burned. Roughly speaking, we burn around 200-600 calories an hour during a brisk walk. So try to walk for around 30-60 minutes a day, or at least 10,000 steps.

CHAPTER SIX: CYCLING

Cycling is another great (and free) activity to add into your new routine, falling into both aerobic and anaerobic camps. Like walking, you can incorporate it into your daily routine so you don't have to carve out extra time for it, if you don't want – for example, by cycling to work. Not only will this add to your exercise quota without you having to make time for it, but you'll save money on fuel or public transport, too.

If you've not been on a bike for a while, or are nervous about taking to the roads, start slowly and with small journeys. When I took up cycling again after a few years of not owning a bike, I was terrified. I lived in London, and back then there weren't many cycle lanes. I left plenty of time to get to work, in case I needed to take a detour, or jump off my bike and walk for a bit to give myself a break. That's the beauty of cycling, you can get on and off your bike anywhere you like! You can build up your confidence slowly. Just like with yoga, try not to compare yourself with other cyclists, who may come zooming past you with total disregard. Let them go at their own pace, and you go at yours.

Cycling burns around 600-800 calories an hour, so if you do it every day, you will have burned plenty of extra calories without thinking too much about it. It's also great for your heart and lungs, and I like to think of it as a daily adventure. Being on a bike feels great – it's free happiness therapy!
If cycling to work isn't an option, maybe go for a long bike ride at the weekend. You'll get to explore different parts of your local

area, and hopefully make new friends along the way. Or take it on the train, as I do, and cycle around the country! Have a look for a local cycling club, if you'd rather be in a group.

CHAPTER SEVEN: DANCING

———

Dancing not only burns calories and and muscle, it releases feel-good chemicals in the brain. It's a low-impact, fun and free way to become healthy and fit – you don't need to go to a class or a club (though they are brilliant), you can put on your favourite music and dance in the comfort of your own home!

Dancing, for me, equals joy. And whatever brings joy, brings health.

Here are some of the other great benefits of dancing:

1. Improves memory and brain functioning whilst learning new steps
2. Sociable and fun
3. Improves cardiovascular health
4. Builds stamina
5. Strengthens bones, muscles and joints
6. Improves coordination
7. Releases endorphins
8. Reduces levels of the stress hormone, cortisol
9. Improves spatial awareness
10. Makes you look and feel super sexy.

CHAPTER EIGHT: TAE BO

Tae Bo has been around since the '90s, and is a series of exercise classes developed and led by American Taekwondo practitioner, Billy Blanks.

It's great for working your abs and upper arms, and if you're looking for definition in those areas, there's not much that will beat it (I've tried).

I used to own all his video cassettes, but now you can buy the DVDs and even take some of the classes for free on YouTube. I can't recommend it enough for getting a really good fitness fix from home. It's high-energy, high-impact, and will leave you grinning from ear to ear.

PART THREE: FEELINGS

CHAPTER NINE: FEELING BAD

When we're overweight and not happy about it, we can feel terrible about ourselves. And when we try and lose weight and don't succeed, or do succeed but then put it back on again, we feel even worse. It can be a depressing cycle to be in.

Also, often one of the reasons we put on weight in the first place is because of how we feel about ourselves or our lives. This might not be an obvious 'self-sabotage' situation, but can be as simple as neglecting to take care of ourselves because we're too busy, or we can't be bothered or we don't feel worthy. There might be something wrong in our lives and we're eating to feel better, more loved, happier, comforted, you name it. How we look is a direct reflection of how we feel about ourselves.

Much of this works together in a symbiotic loop. If you feel bad about yourself, you're more likely to eat rubbish and not exercise. And if you gain weight, you're more likely to feel bad about yourself.

Sometimes you also put on weight or eat the wrong things because you're trying to numb yourself or 'stuff down' feelings. These can be so uncomfortable that you'll do anything not to feel them. Maybe it's due to something bad that's happened, or a lack of self worth, the end of a relationship, a lack of direction in life, boredom, general dissatisfaction, carelessness or even trauma.

You don't need anyone's permission to turn over a new leaf and start afresh. This is your life. Just because you've done something one way doesn't mean you can't change and do it another way. That's what's so great about life – you wake up each morning and get another shot at it. We can completely change our own story. All it takes is a paradigm shift.

Of course you must acknowledge where, if any, deep-seated problems lie, and get to the root cause (there may be more than one) to heal it by seeking professional help. But a lot of the work can be done on your own.

Getting to the bottom of why you do what you do, and why you feel what you feel, is VITAL. Only you have the power and choice to make a change. And you need to ask yourself if you're willing to do what it takes today, and for the rest of your life. Only you can do this.

CHAPTER TEN: JOURNALING

———————

Keeping a journal can be a great way of measuring your progress, as well as monitoring how you feel about things. Getting it all out on paper each day is very cathartic, and also serves as a reminder of how far you've come and what you were going through at the time so you can look back and appreciate the journey.

What gets measured gets done, so use your notebook to jot down everything you ate, how much sleep you got, and what exercise you took each day – if you use a fitness app you can add in times and stats. I recommend not weighing yourself until you are at least 2-3 months into this new routine, but some people find it helpful to keep a record of their weight. Up to you.

Find a quiet place each day to write about your thoughts and feelings. Try and explain why things are the way they are and what you intend to do about it. I find that doing this in the early morning on awakening, or in the evening, is most helpful. I always write about how I feel – it really helps get it all off my chest. And at least if nobody else is there to bear witness, at least the page is.

The more you get used to carving out quiet time for reflection, the healthier your body and mind will be.

As this book is about simplifying, streamlining and getting back to basics, perhaps think about a few things that you can eliminate from your life – things that cause you stress, harm, anxiety, upset or unnecessary suffering. If you apply the 80/20 rule, what are the 20% of things, people, situations, foods and habits that cause you 80% of the problems or damage? Can you get rid of some of that 20%? Removing things and having a clearout will free up space in our lives and our bodies, and allow better, more nurturing things in. Then we can flow again. Have a look at the book *Essentialism* for some inspiration.

CHAPTER ELEVEN: GOAL-SETTING

What do you want to do with the rest of your life? And more importantly, who do you want to become?

Taking some time to figure out the answers to those questions can often help shift things in your mind, body and life.

When you know your 'Big Why' – the reason you do what you do, and what's most important to you – you have direction and purpose.

It can also be useful to have those questions written down to look at first thing in the morning when you're doing your meditation or morning walk and your mind is clear. Taking a few moments to ask yourself where you're going and how you can become a better person is a great way to start the day.

By getting clear in our heads, our bodies will also follow suit, and our subconscious mind can then help us get there.

What we focus on, we get more of. So by training our brains to focus on a positive outcome, we are helping ourselves instead of sabotaging or hindering ourselves. Often we can be our own worst enemy, and don't even know why we do the things we do. Our habits are so ingrained they've become second nature – what is comfortable isn't necessarily right. The brain is programmed to like what's familiar and to keep us safe. It's not programmed to make good choices for us or to make us happy.

Reprogramming our subconscious mind through imagination and visualisation takes time and effort but will absolutely be worth it in the end.

TOP TIP: What gets measured gets done, so take a few minutes now to write down exactly how you want to be looking, feeling and what you want to be doing in 6-12 months' time. Describe in detail an ideal scene.

If you imagine you're wearing beautiful new clothes and are looking healthy and glowing, with good friends and/or the love of your life, really intensify those feelings so they sink into your bones. Write about this ideal scene now.

It can sometimes also be helpful to cut out pictures of things you'd like to be doing, or an outfit you'd like to fit into. You can also find these pictures online and save them to your desktop or phone so you see them regularly. Focus on those feelings and those pictures as often as you can, making sure you're not focusing on the feeling of 'lack' or 'gap' between now and then – only the end result as if it's true now. Feel it on a cellular level. This is where change occurs.

CHAPTER TWELVE: MEDITATION

Find a quiet place each day to spend a few minutes alone. Some people like to sit cross-legged, but you can just as easily lie down or take a walk. I like to do this first thing in the morning as soon as I've woken up. Taking a few minutes to sit calmly is a powerful way to start the day. You regain control and clarity.

I then take a walk in nature (but any walk is a good walk!) and think about things. I try and think of all the things I like about my life and what I'm grateful for. But my mind inevitably wanders to all sorts, and that's OK too. Creating thinking time is one of the best ways to live a sane, purposeful life. If you don't have time to think, how do you know you're OK and on track?

It's important to tend to ourselves, and our mental health is as important as our physical health. In fact, the two are very closely interlinked, so when we take care of one, we're also taking care of the other.

Every morning and every evening for the next six months, I'd like you to set your timer and sit for 10 minutes in a quiet place and focus on your breathing and on calming your mind. Place a hand on your heart or stomach and breath quietly. Never underestimate the power of this one simple exercise.

QUICK MEDITATION

1. Sit or lie down or start walking
2. For the first few seconds, take deep, purposeful breaths
3. As you're taking these breaths, say in your mind "let go, let go" in a calm voice
4. Let any thoughts pop up and float on without getting involved emotionally, keep letting go
5. Now in your mind think of a garden, and as you breathe, imagine you are surrounded by trees and flowers
6. Continue for as long as you can and enjoy the peace.

CHAPTER THIRTEEN: EFT / TAPPING

Thought Field Therapy (TFT) – or "tapping", as it's known – may seem like an odd thing to do at first, but it's hugely effective, and scientifically proven to work. Invented by American psychologist Roger Callahan, it stimulates the meridian points in the body, and can relieve pain, desperation, trauma, anxiety and any urges. It's deceptively simple, but once you've mastered the sequence, you can use it anytime, any place.

It's ideal for when you feel anxious, afraid, stressed, hyper, angry or like eating something unhealthy or sabotaging your new lifestyle in another way.

TOP TIP:
Sometimes it's enough to just tap your fingers together or tap on your chest. Also, if you're not in a place where you can do your tapping physically, you can do it in your head instead – it works just as well. Our nervous systems can't tell the difference between a real and vividly imagined event, and we can use this to our advantage here.

Here is the sequence as I learned it. You can do it on your right or left side, using your right or left hand.

1. Rate how you're feeling on a scale of 1-10, with 10 being the worst or most acute

2. Repeat the following phrase out loud, filling in the blanks: "Even though I feel ___, I deeply and profoundly love and accept myself." Repeat this phrase three times while tapping on the side of your hand, at the karate chop point

3. Now focus on the negative situation or emotion as you run through the following sequence

4. Pat the top of your head 10 times with your hand

5. Tap just above your eyebrow 10 times with the tips of your index and middle fingers

6. Tap just below your eye 10 times

7. Tap above your lip 10 times, and below your bottom lip 10 times

8. Using your hand, pat under your arm 10 times, around four inches beneath your armpit. If you're a woman, it's right where your bra strap is

9. Tap on your collarbone, at the base of your neck

10. Then use both hands to gently tap around the chest area. Keep breathing, and keep focused on the negative feeling

11. Tap on the tip of your index finger

12. Tap on your collarbone again

13. Tap all fingers together

14. Now tap on the back of your hand on the "gamut spot", between your little finger and ring finger. While you're doing this, continue with the other steps

15. Close your eyes then open them again. Look down to the right then down to the left. Roll your eyes clockwise then anticlockwise then close them again. Keep focused on the problem. Don't let your mind wander!

16. Hum the first part of a song, eg "Happy Birthday", which activates the right side of the brain, then count out loud from 1-5, which activates the left

17. Keep tapping on the back of your hand, between your fingers. Take a deep breath. Hum Happy Birthday again
18. Tap under the eye 10 times, and under your arm 10 times, then under your collarbone again.
19. Repeat the phrase: "I deeply and profoundly love and accept myself."

Take a deep breath and notice how you feel. How would you rate it out of 10? You should have reduced your negative feeling considerably. Repeat the exercise as many times as necessary to bring the feeling right down to a 1 or 2 out of 10.

CHAPTER FOURTEEN: R&R

It's so important to rest well and give the body the recovery time it needs. If we're not well rested, everything else is out of balance, and life feels so much less manageable. Our mind starts to play tricks on us, we remember things differently, we have less patience, and our body is under stress – and that's when problems start to build up.

When the body's in 'sympathetic' fight, flight or freeze mode, a cocktail of hormones course through it so we can deal with the threatening situation. In 'parasympathetic' rest and digest mode, our body is at ease and can process, grow and heal. Think about how an antelope runs for its life when it's being chased by a lion. Then once it's out of danger, it goes straight back to grazing and relaxing again as if nothing happened.

Making sure you're getting enough rest and sleep gives you time to recuperate, recalibrate, rest and digest. If you're always in fight or flight mode, your body will take a battering, your immune system will be seriously impaired and it will be very difficult to be truly healthy and happy. Sleep is of prime importance, so get as much as you possibly can.

Rest can mean meditation – even 5-10 minutes of sitting quietly with your eyes closed – or lying down on the carpet starting at the ceiling, contemplating life while looking out of the window, reading a book (watching television or looking at a screen doesn't count) or taking a bath. You get the idea. If you're not used to this kind of non-activity, buy a book or take a course in mindful meditation to start you off. It takes a bit of practice, but will absolutely change your life.

Create a cool, dark, comfortable bedroom where you're not to be disturbed each night. Take a look at your bed and see what improvements can be made to ensure you get the best possible sleep you can.

Back in the 1950s, we used to get an average of eight hours' sleep a night. These days, it's more like five. According to recent research, only around 7% of the UK population get enough sleep. In America this is just 4%.

A lack of sleep has been linked to overeating and weight gain, so getting enough quality sleep is vital to being healthy and in good shape. It also makes us feel calmer and able to think creatively and remember things.

Insomnia, or poor-quality sleep, not only impairs judgement and mental health, it dramatically affects our appetite and weight. It interferes with our metabolism and hormones associated with hunger and feeling full. It also contributes to stress, which means we often reach for the wrong foods in order to comfort ourselves[27]. All in all, not getting enough sleep is disastrous for our health, so make sure you get at least your full eight hour quota each night.

It's important to note that underlying health problems can affect both sleep and the ability to lose weight, so if this applies to you, these must be tackled first and foremost by seeking medical help.

Journaling about your day before bed can be a good way to unwind before bed. So can taking a warm bath with magnesium

---

[27] https://www.nhs.uk/news/obesity/sleep-affects-weight-loss/

salts or Epsom salts and some essential oils, pop on some relaxing music, light a few candles and chill out.

Looking after ourselves requires a great deal of effort – it's not easy, by any stretch – but it sends a powerful signal to our brains that we love ourselves and are worthwhile creatures, and this in turn helps us make positive choices for ourselves – choices that support us rather than sabotage us. It all works in a feedback loop.

CHAPTER FIFTEEN: GRATITUDE

Just as it's important to be physically healthy, it's important to be emotionally and spiritually healthy, too. A gratitude journal is a really good way to build your happiness muscle.

Each night, I'd like you to write down (or think about in your head) 10 things you are grateful for about your life and about the day that has just passed. These can be as little or as big as you like. The most important thing is that you feel really good about them. Really enjoy each one as you go through them. Express thanks for your family, friends, home, the work you do, the big and little moments that have pleased you throughout the day.

By focusing on the positives rather than the negatives, our subconscious mind gets reprogrammed to bring more positive things to it. Like attracts like.

Keeping a gratitude journal is so simple, yet is extremely powerful. As with everything else in this book, it's a tried-and-tested method of bringing more health and positivity into your life.

CHAPTER SIXTEEN: SELF IMAGE

It's easy to view ourselves in a less-than-favourable light. We can be our own worst enemy sometimes. But our perception of ourselves is hugely important if we want to change the way we look and feel. Thoughts and feelings fuel behaviour and behaviour fuels thoughts and feelings.

Negative emotions and mindset, poor self-image, boredom, feeling lost, trapped, unloved, stressed and depressed all contribute to weight gain, disease and ill health. Fixing your mindset is a surefire way to come back to health. But it takes time.

For the sake of this exercise, I'd like you to write down 10 things you love about yourself. Try and mix up physical and other characteristics. By feeling grateful for our bodies, we stop hating it and start loving it. The change will be slow but subtle.

Think about your favourite feature – is it your eyes, nose, stomach, legs? Give love and thanks for that feature. When we look for the things we like about our body instead of the things we don't like or wish we could change, we start to turn a corner into a realm of loving ourselves instead of hating ourselves. This change can be slow or fast, it's up to you. The more you practice it, the quicker the change will be. But each day, come up with at least 10 things you really like about your body, and for each one say thank you.
You can also say thank you for your eyes, ears, heart, stomach, kidneys, liver, spine, skin, legs, etc. Because your body and mind

are closely interlinked, when you focus on those areas you are happy about, your body responds by giving you more things to be happy about.

Once you're done, stick that list in a place you'll see it every day, such as your fridge or in your wallet.

For extra power, you can read this list out loud in front of the mirror each day. This might seem silly at first, but stick with it. The more we repeat these statements and affirmations, the more power they have. Give thanks for the body that has carried you through life up until this point. It's pretty amazing. Focus on the things you don't like or can't change, and you will get more of the same.

Look in the mirror and say to yourself, "I am enough". Repeat this at least 10 times a day.

Whoever you are, whatever size or shape you are, be grateful, love yourself, nurture yourself and accept yourself and miracles will occur.

A lot of our confidence and self-esteem comes from how we behave towards ourselves, the way we talk about ourselves in our heads and the way we describe ourselves to others. Never, ever use negative language when describing yourself or your body.

Self talk becomes a self-fulfilling prophecy. Studies have shown that words carry a frequency that affects our cells. This is why it's very important to speak positively, and not beat yourself up. If you love your body, rather than hate it, it actually begins to listen – much like a child.

Our body responds obediently to our thoughts, ideas and beliefs. If we see ourselves as fat, ugly, old, depressed, or in any kind of negative light, that is how our body will respond. Argue for your limitations, and they're yours. So stop all negative self-talk and criticism, either out loud or in your head. You wouldn't talk to your best friend that way, so don't talk to yourself like that.

Find role models of people you'd like to emulate or look like, and instead of focusing on your differences, try and emulate them. How would they move their body? How would they think about themselves? What habits and routines would they have? Keep those pictures somewhere you'll see regularly. If you like you can spend a few minutes each day with your eyes closed visualising yourself in a different body and enjoy how that feels. Take as much time as you can with this exercise, and really immerse yourself in the experience.

Our bodies and minds are highly suggestible, so when you truly believe something, or when you think or feel it with conviction, it often starts to become true.

In NLP, this technique is called 'modelling' – stepping into the shoes of someone you want to emulate. It's incredibly powerful.

The power of belief is so strong that studies have shown that people can change their physiology just by how they talk, act and perceive themselves. In one experiment – 'Counterclockwise' by Harvard psychologist Ellen Langer – a group of eight elderly men were taken on a retreat for a week to see if they could reverse the signs of ageing. Everything about the place they stayed in was designed to look like 20 years earlier, and the subjects were asked to behave as if the year was also 20 years earlier. Within just one week, all men were tested and had "youthed' considerably, even playing a touch football game on the front lawn on the last day.

The subconscious mind is like a heat-seeking missile. Programme it right, and it's amazing where it can take you.

Another example is of a man who was told by his doctor that he had terminal cancer and had six months to live. Sure enough, six months later he died. Sadly, after the event, it was discovered that his medical records had been mixed up with someone else's. He was completely healthy. He died of false conviction and belief. This is why doctors giving patients survival timeframes and percentage life expectancies can actually be really damaging.

Your mind and body are connected more than you possibly realise. Use your thoughts, beliefs and behaviour very wisely. Analyse them, reassess them, and make sure they are serving you not killing you.

It's widely accepted that 30 per cent of patients who take a dummy painkiller actually experience pain relief as if a real tablet has been taken. Sometimes that figure is nudging the same as that for the actual drug – the placebo effect is so strong.

The good news is that the power is within you. Not just at the behavioural level, but at the conscious level. You have consciousness and intelligence running through every cell – think about yourself in a new light, and that light will be yours.

You have the power to make a change – and it can happen as quickly as you want it to. In just one year, 98 per cent of your body's atoms will be completely new. So the body you have now will be a different body in 12 months' time. The stomach lining replenishes itself every 5-7 days, the skin once a month, and the skeleton every three months. This gives you immense opportunity to sculpt and recreate yourself however you wish. The cells in your body listen to every single thing you say, think or feel about yourself, even if you're not necessarily aware of it consciously. Your body listens and obeys your commands.

Another good idea is to give yourself a 'rebrand'. Look at the clothes that aren't working for you, and throw away anything that makes you feel less than amazing. If you can afford to, buy a few new items, and get a new haircut. Giving our image a rebrand signals a new start to the brain, and to those around us. You could also change your perfume/aftershave, and pay a visit to a spa or beauty salon to get some pampering and grooming in.

Once you start taking these small steps towards re-creating your self image, the snowball effect will kick in. Don't wait for the time when you're at your ideal weight to do this. Start now, and it will feed into the new version of yourself in your own mind.

Conclusion

That's it! By now I hope you are feeling happier and healthier in yourself, and more vibrant in your body and life. Eat well and sleep well and nearly everything else will fall into place.

Remember to fill your life with things that are meaningful to you. Things that make you come alive. Feed your brain and your soul only the very best. Seek fulfilment. The more you do this, the less likely you are to eat rubbish and the more your body will change. And if your body changes, your mind changes and your life changes.

I hope this book has helped you. If you've enjoyed it, please do leave me an honest review on Amazon. I've also released a 30-day fitness journal and a 30-day healthy eating journal.

If you would like more personalised help, just email me on the address below.

I wish you all the health, happiness, peace, strength, success and – of course – love in the world. Thank you for being here.

Love,
A.C Miller

acmillerbooks@gmail.com
https://acmillerbooks.wordpress.com

RESOURCES

Books

Atomic Habits by James Clear

Becoming Raw by Brenda Davis

Becoming Vegan by Brenda Davis

Dr Clark's Healthy Recipes by Hulda Regehr Clark

Foods That Harm, Foods That Heal by Reader's Digest

Health Magic Through Chlorophyll From Living Plant Life by Bernard Jensen

How Not to Die by Dr Michael Greger

How to Go Vegan by Veganuary

Ikigai by Héctor Garcia and Fransesc Miralles

Proteinaholic by Garth Davis MD

The China Study by T.Colin Campbell

The Cure For All Diseases by Hulda Regehr Clark

The Raw Foods Bible by Craig B. Sommers

Vegan Planet by Robin Robertson

Whole by T. Colin Campbell

Your Best Year Yet by Jinny Ditzler

Websites

Proteinaholic: www.proteinaholic.com/

The Vegan Society: www.vegansociety.com/

One Green Planet: www.onegreenplanet.org/

Oxygen Advantage: www.oxygenadvantage.com

Yoga With Adriene: www.yogawithadriene.com

Paul McKenna: www.paulmckenna.com

Tae Bo: www.taebo.com

Find What Feels Good yoga downloads: www.fwfg.com

ABOUT A.C MILLER

A.C Miller is a travel, health and psychology writer based in London, England. Her other books include *Reboot* and *The Heartbreak Cure*, as well as notebooks and journals to help people achieve health and wellness.

www.ingramcontent.com/pod-product-compliance
Lightning Source LLC
Chambersburg PA
CBHW050050260726
48658CB00005B/1870